IAMSE Manuals

The book series IAMSE Manuals is established to rapidly deploy the latest developments and best evidence-based examples in medical education, offering all who teach in healthcare the most current information to succeed in their task by publishing short "how-to-guides" on a variety of topics relevant to medical teaching. The series aims to make the best and latest evidence-based methods for teaching in medical education to educators around the world, to improve the quality of teaching in healthcare education, and to establish greater interest in the teaching of the medical sciences.

More information about this series at http://www.springer.com/series/16034

Ruth E. Levine • Patricia D. Hudes

How-to Guide for Team-Based Learning

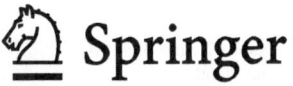 Springer

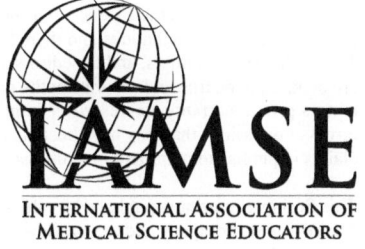

Ruth E. Levine
Psychiatry and Behavioral Sciences
The University of Texas Medical Branch
Galveston, TX, USA

Patricia D. Hudes
Academic Affairs/Community Health
Wright State University
Dayton, OH, USA

Previously self-published by IAMSE; under ISBN 978-1-4675-6665-0.

IAMSE Manuals
ISBN 978-3-030-62922-9   ISBN 978-3-030-62923-6   (eBook)
https://doi.org/10.1007/978-3-030-62923-6

This Springer imprint is published by the registered company Springer Nature Switzerland AG
The registered company address is: Gewerbestrasse 11, 6330 Cham, Switzerland

Photo Credits

Photos in this manual were taken by Darren Harbert in the Spring of 2012, during a TBL session designed and facilitated by Dr. Osvaldo Lopez for the Wright State University Boonshoft School of Medicine class of 2015.

Purpose

The purpose of this guide is to:

1. Provide an overview of the fundamental components of Team-Based Learning (TBL) and its advantages over conventional instructional methods.
2. Serve as a blueprint for instructors who wish to begin teaching TBL in a course or curriculum.
3. Identify factors that will facilitate or sabotage a successful implementation of TBL.
4. Provide additional resources to learn the knowledge and skills to start a TBL program.

Contents

About the Authors

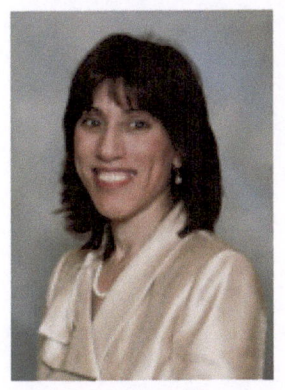

Ruth E. Levine, MD is the Clarence Ross Miller Professor of Psychiatry in the Department of Psychiatry and Behavioral Sciences and the Associate Dean for Student Affairs and Admissions Dean for at the University of Texas Medical Branch in Galveston, Texas, where she has served on the faculty for 30 years. She was also the inaugural director for UTMB's Academy of Master Teachers, established in 2006. Dr. Levine has established Team-Based Learning courses in undergraduate and graduate medical education settings and has provided workshops and consultative services for numerous health science faculty nationally and internationally. She has authored and co-edited a variety of publications on Team-Based Learning including co-editing the text *Team-Based Learning in Health Professions Education*. (Stylus 2008)

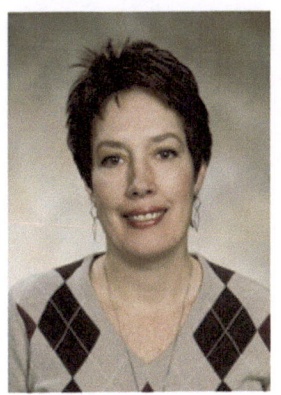

Patricia D. Hudes, MSIT is the director of Faculty Development at the Boonshoft School of Medicine, in Dayton, Ohio, where she has worked since 2002. Her main goal is to promote teaching and learning experiences that focus on self-direct, active, and lifelong learning. She is an Instructional Designer; therefore, a strong believer that for learning experiences to be meaningful and effective, they have to be carefully crafted, following a systematic instructional design process, and based on solid pedagogical principles. She has provided workshops and consultations related to medical education and has co-authored several publications on Team-Based Learning.

Chapter 1
What is Team-Based Learning?

1.1 Advantages Over Conventional Instructional Methods

1.1.1 Focus on Application of Knowledge

Team-Based Learning™ (TBL) is an active learning strategy that focuses on application of knowledge through a sequence of events that include individual work, teamwork and immediate feedback.

Dr. Larry Michaelsen first developed TBL in the 1970s while teaching at the University of Oklahoma Business School when his classes increased in size from 40 to 120. Recognizing that large group lectures were inherently ineffective in motivating students to engage and immerse themselves in higher-level problem solving, Dr. Michaelsen crafted TBL to help students become more active and involved in their learning.

TBL was adopted by undergraduate teachers in business and science education, and was later introduced to health science education in approximately 2001 [1, 2]. Team-Based Learning is now used worldwide by instructors in numerous schools of medicine, nursing, dentistry, pharmacy, and other health science disciplines.

1.1.2 Positive Learning Outcomes

Active learning strategies in general and TBL in particular have been associated with a variety of positive learning outcomes. Team-Based Learning in medical education has been associated with increased engagement within the classroom, increased appreciation of the value of teams by students, and acquisition of knowledge as good as and, in some cases, better than conventional didactic methods [3]. Literature suggests that TBL can improve student performance, especially in academically weaker students [4, 5].

© The Author(s), under exclusive license to Springer Nature Switzerland AG 2021
R. E. Levine, P. D. Hudes, *How-to Guide for Team-Based Learning*, IAMSE
Manuals, https://doi.org/10.1007/978-3-030-62923-6_1

1.2   TBL Steps

Every TBL module or unit of instruction consists of a basic 3-step process as is illustrated in Fig. 1.1. This includes:

1. **Pre-class Preparation**
2. **Readiness Assurance**
3. **Application of Key Concepts**

1.2.1   Step 1: Pre-class Preparations

The pre-class preparation is assigned to the students and consists of information they need to master to meet the learning objectives. The information may include book chapters, learning guides, online modules, research articles, or even face-to-face learning sessions such as lectures or labs. Lectures can be delivered live or can be recorded and made available before a TBL class. Students are expected to review and be prepared to utilize the information during the TBL in class session.

Instructors need to be very specific and precise when assigning preparatory material. If excessive or inappropriate material is assigned, students will become frustrated or arrive to the TBL session unprepared.

Step 1 Pre-Class Preparation (out-of-class)	**Prepare for TBL Module** Students study independently in preparation for the in-class TBL sessions			
	Assure Readiness for Application Exercises Students master key concepts			
	IRAT Individual Readiness Assurance Test	**GRAT** Group Readiness Assurance Test	**Appeals**	**Discussion**
Step 2 Readiness Assurance (in-class)	Individual students complete a short multiple-choice test based on the key concepts from the advance assignment.	Teams of 5-7 students re-take the same test, and recieve immediate feedback regarding their answer choices.	Teams may submit written appeals to any questions that were missed on the GRAT. This is an open-book process - teams must work together to create a cogent argument for appeal.	Class discusses any questions or concepts that need clarification.
Step 3 Application of Key Concepts (in-class)	**Apply Key Concepts** Students apply key concepts: teams collaborate on in-class application assignments aimed at developing students' higher-level cognitive skills. The application exercises are characterized by the "4 Ss" (Significant Problem, Same Problem, Specific Choice, and Simultaneous Report).			

Fig. 1.1 TBL steps

The primary principle of pre-class preparation is that the material is assigned to the student before the TBL session begins, and the student will be held responsible for knowledge of the material once the TBL session starts. The pre-class preparation materials should be accompanied by specific and clear learning objectives.

1.2.2   Step 2: Readiness Assurance

Readiness assurance consists of four steps:

- Individual readiness assurance test (IRAT)
- Group or Team readiness assurance test (GRAT)
- Appeals
- Facilitator feedback or clarification

1.2.2.1   Individual Readiness Assurance Test (IRAT)

The principle of readiness assurance is to make sure that all learners have mastered the pre-class material so that they will be ready for the higher-level problem solving that is part of the application assignments.

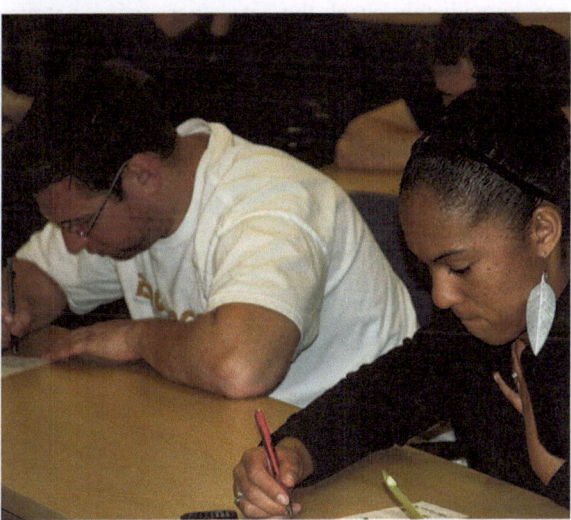

In the first part of readiness assurance, students take a short quiz or "individual readiness assurance test" (IRAT). The IRAT questions are typically multiple- choice and intended to enable the instructor to assess whether the students have mastered the key concepts from the pre-class preparation [6]. IRATs should be well written and derived from foundational material. Items should not be picky or based on trivial facts from the readings. Poorly written IRATs will frustrate and anger students and can sabotage an otherwise good TBL module.

Confidence testing is a strategy that is recommended when administering IRATs. Confidence testing operates as follows: each item is worth 2–4 points. Students are instructed to assign the number of points to their chosen answer based on how confident or prepared they are when choosing their answer. For example, in an IRAT in which items are worth 4 points each, a student who is very confident that the answer to "Question #1" is "A" may assign 4 points to "A." Another student who may be torn between the choice of "A" and "B" may assign 2 points to "A" and 2 points to "B."

Instructor can distribute scantrons to students in which "Question #1" is assigned numbers 1–4 on the scantron. Students who want to assign all 4 points to "A" would fill in "A" 4 times in the scantron, and students who would want to fill in "A" twice could do so, and then fill in "B" twice as well.

Confidence testing helps students quantify how prepared they feel before they begin the group portion of the readiness assurance process. It is a useful cognitive step for students to negotiate during the team portion of readiness assurance.

1.2.2.2   Group or Team Readiness Assurance Test (GRAT)

Once IRAT answer sheets are collected, students are prompted to join their teams and take the exact same test as a team. Students should agree on the answers to each question and then immediately check the correctness using a strategy such as the Immediate Feedback Assessment Technique (IF-AT). As teams agree upon a consensus choice, learners "scratch off" the portion of the IF-AT corresponding to that choice. Visit the Epstein Educational Enterprises website (www.epsteineducation. com) for more information (Fig. 1.2). If a team scratches the correct choice, a star is revealed and the team earns points. The team is rewarded with higher points for a correct answer on the first try, and lower points for each subsequent try.

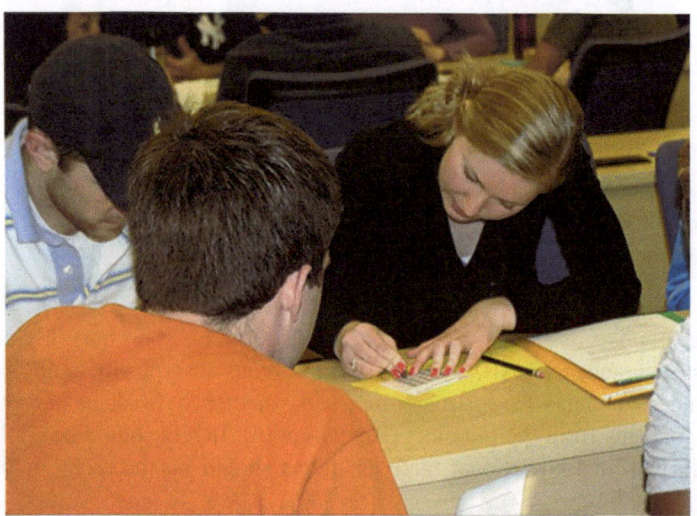

IMMEDIATE FEEDBACK ASSESSMENT TECHNIQUE (IF AT®)

Name _____   Test # _____

Subject _____   Total _____

SCRATCH OFF COVERING TO EXPOSE ANSWER

	A	B	C	D	Score
1.				★	____
2.	☐	★			____
3.					____
4.					____
5.					____
6.					____
7.					____
8.					

Fig. 1.2 IF-AT—Immediate feedback assessment technique

Teams should arrive at an agreement and check each answer one at a time since the immediate and continuous feedback derived from this process rapidly facilitates the process of team development.

New instructors often ask how many and how difficult RAT questions should be. Readiness assurance questions should include a balance of fundamental items that all prepared students can easily answer, along with challenging items that require the talent of the entire team. Students will be discouraged if they are given too many RATs or too many items, or the questions are too tricky or difficult. Conversely, a RAT that is not sufficiently challenging will not reinforce pre-class preparation or assist in the process of team building.

Some new instructors become enamored with the engagement generated by GRATs and spend too much of the TBL time on readiness assurance. Instructors should remember that the essence of TBL comes from the application of key concepts and that readiness assurance is only an intermediary step to ensure that students are ready for that third and most crucial component.

1.2.2.3 Appeals

Once teams complete the GRAT they can post their scores for whole class viewing. Posting group scores helps teams gain perspective about the relative difficulty of the RAT and also facilitates team building. Posting also reminds slower teams to pick up the pace so as not to delay the progress of the entire class. Teams then have the opportunity to return to the pre-class preparation materials and review items missed on the GRAT.

Teams may appeal a grade if they believe that an item was either scored incorrectly or poorly constructed. To appeal an item the team believes was scored incorrectly, teams must produce written evidence, usually from the source material, citing the reasons they believe their answer was correct and the instructor's answer was incorrect. To appeal an item the team believes was poorly constructed, the team must re-write the item and submit the new item as the appeal.

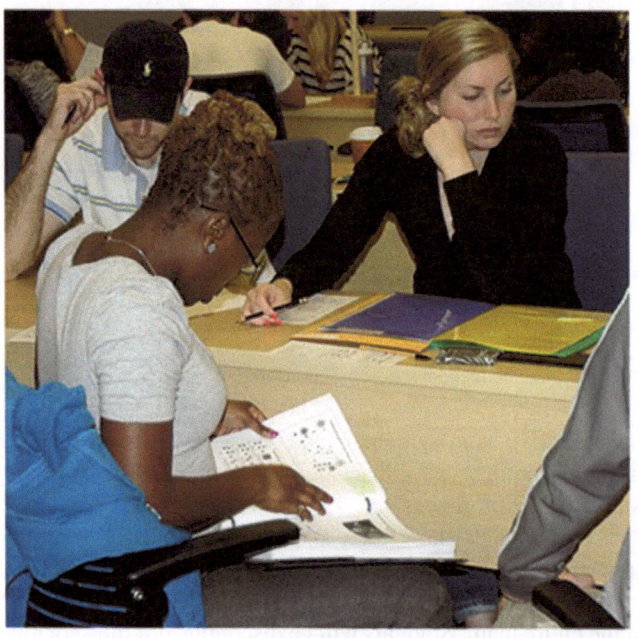

The rules for appeals include that the team (not a single member of the team) must initiate the appeal and that the appeal must be argued in writing, generally with documentation. In most instances, only the team that appeals an item will be given credit for a successful appeal. The appeal's purpose is to motivate teams to review material that they missed during the GRAT, and thus clarify their understanding of the information they will need during the application phase of the TBL module.

1.2.2.4   Facilitator Feedback or Clarification

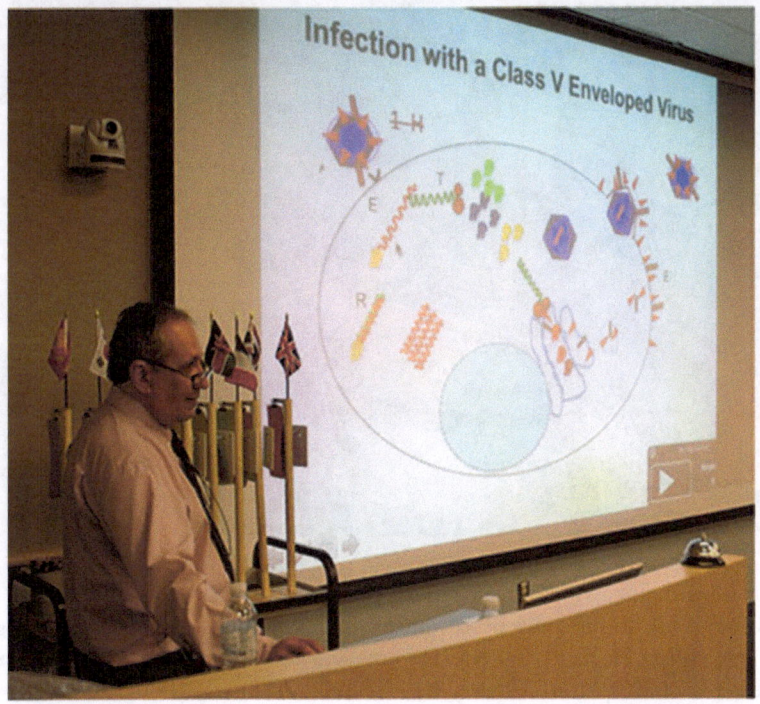

The last component of readiness assurance involves a review of the RAT and discussion of any items that remain a source of confusion for the students. Some facilitators may find it useful to conduct a "mini-lecture" during this period of time in order to ensure that the key principles from the pre-class preparation materials are understood by all of the learners.

It is useful for the facilitator to circulate among the teams during the GRAT portion of readiness assurance so that he/she can hear what concepts require the most time for team discussion. Items requiring the most team discussion usually provide the most fruitful topics for the facilitator feedback portion of readiness assurance. Even when the teams do very well on their GRATs several topics typically still require clarification.

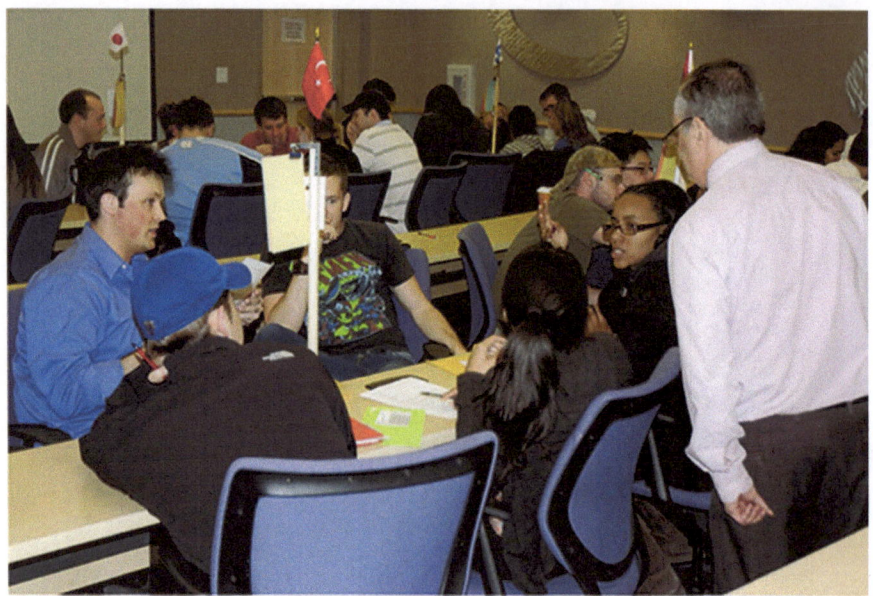

Some instructors will ask teams to choose and post on the board one to two RAT items they wish to have discussed during the clarification period. Prompting the students to select the most challenging items will enable the teams and the instructor to better plan the topics of discussion.

1.2.3   Step 3: Application of Key Concepts

The final step of TBL is application of key concepts, in which teams engage in real life problem solving. Applications are ideally problems that are so challenging that they require the knowledge and skills of the entire team to solve. The application exercises can take many forms, but all are characterized by the "4 Ss":

- *Significant Problem*
- *Same Problem*
- *Specific Choice*
- *Simultaneous Report*

Significant Problem: All problems must be of significance to the learner. In order to be significant, problems must be relevant to what the learner sees himself or herself doing in the future. For example, a pharmacy student must see an application as relevant to helping her to be a better pharmacist. TBL problems must be about doing not just about knowing.

Same Problem: All teams must work on the same problem at the same time. The reason working on the same problem is important is that only by having the whole class focused on the same issue will everyone remain engaged when that one problem is discussed.

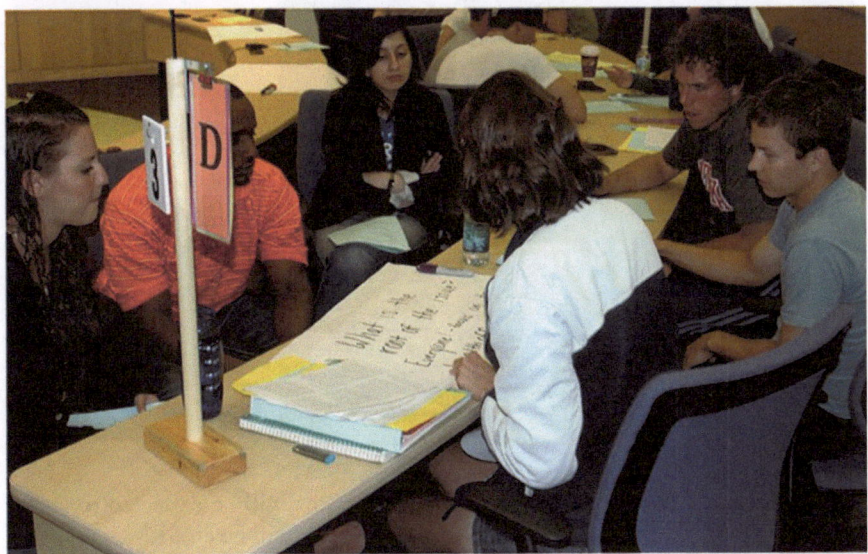

Specific Choice: Each problem must have a specific solution, or "specific choice" as an answer. In some cases, problems will be structured like multiple-choice questions, but in other instances teams will be prompted to create their own "specific choice." For example, teams may be given white boards and asked to write out a differential diagnosis for a clinical presentation, but then circle the most likely diagnosis. In another instance, teams may be prompted to design a complex experiment, post the experiment on the wall, and then do a "gallery walk" in which they examine all of the other teams' experiments. Teams will then be prompted to make a "specific choice" in which they must choose the best experiment, with the caveat that they are not allowed to vote for their own.

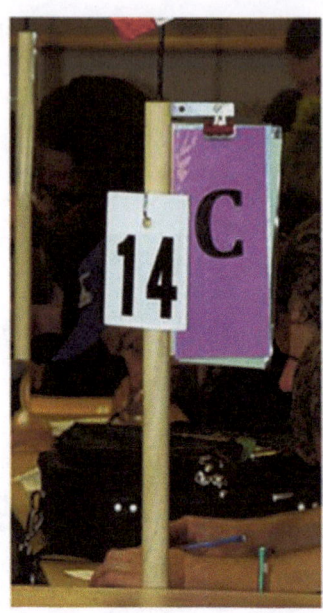

Simultaneous Report: When prompted, all teams will be expected to reveal their choices at the same time, so that the entire class will be able to see what the other teams have chosen. Simultaneous report can occur a variety of ways, including displaying flash cards (numbered or lettered) or using Audience Response System 'clickers.' Simultaneous reporting generates both engagement and accountability.

During the application phase, the facilitator poses application problems to the teams. The teams should spend considerable time discussing different options before arriving at a "specific choice," and revealing their choice to the whole class (at the same time as the other teams reveal their choices). The facilitator subsequently moderates a "whole class" discussion in which he/she facilitates an "inter-team" discussion of the problems. Sometimes the teams will hold up lettered or numbered cards corresponding to their choices; at other times they will post complex solutions, compare and contrast each other's work, and simultaneously vote on the best solution, or vote on a ranking of the best solutions. The best application exercises will yield vigorous and engaging debates revealing a sophisticated understanding of the course concepts.

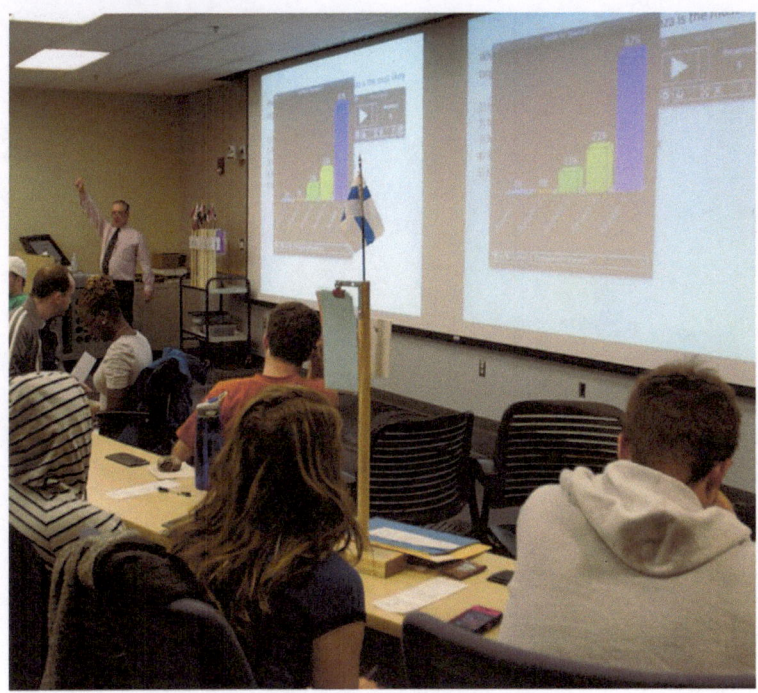

References

1. Haidet P, O'Malley KJ, Richards B. An initial experience with "team learning" in medical education. Acad Med. 2002;77:40–4.
2. Searle NS, Haidet P, Kelly PA, Schneider VF, Seidel CL, Richards BF. Team learning in medical education: experiences at ten institutions. Acad Med. 2003;78(10 suppl):S55–8.
3. Levine RE, O'Boyle M, Haidet P, Lynn DJ, Stone MM, Wolf DV, Paniagua FA. Transforming a clinical clerkship with team learning. Teach Learn Med. 2004;16:270–5.
4. Chung EK, Rhee JA, Baik YH, Oh-Sun A. The effect of team-based learning in medical ethics education. Med Teach. 2009;31:1013–7.
5. Koles P, Stolfi A, Borges N, Nelson S, Parmelee D. The impact of team-based learning on medical students' academic performance. Acad Med. 2010;85(11):1739–45.
6. Michaelsen LK, Parmelee DX, McMahon KK, Levine RE. Team-Based Learning for Health Professions Education: A Guide to Using Small Groups for Improving Learning. Chapter 2. Sterling, VA: Stylus; 2008.

Chapter 2
How to Design and Implement TBL

2.1 Backward Design

Designing a TBL course or curriculum is best accomplished using the principles of Backward Design [1]. To understand Backward Design, consider how courses are usually created:

For a 12-week course:

- Find a textbook
- Divide the text book into 12 sections
- Assign readings (one section of readings per week)
- Create lectures to accompany the readings (one to three lectures per week, depending on the course)
- Deliver the lectures
- Write an exam over the lectures and the readings
- Administer an end of course exam
- If some pesky administrator asks for objectives—write objectives to go with the course and turn them in after everything is organized.

The principle of Backward Design posits that a course should be designed the other way around: you start with the learning objectives, followed by the creation of assessments that meet the objectives and finally create the materials that will support learning. When creating a TBL module, the instructor should use the Backward Design process as follows:

1. **Situational Factors**
   Consider the situational factors that will be impacting your course: Who are the learners? At what level are they in the curriculum? What other courses are they taking? What are their competencies and expectations?

R. E. Levine, P. D. Hudes, *How-to Guide for Team-Based Learning*, IAMSE
Manuals, https://doi.org/10.1007/978-3-030-62923-6_2

2. **Learning Objectives**

What are your objectives for the course? And for a TBL module, specifically, what do you want your learners to DO as a result of the TBL session?

3. **Assessment Activities**

How will you assess your learners? (These are the application exercises). How will you make sure your learners are ready for assessment? (This is the readiness assurance process)

4. **Learning Materials**

What learning materials do you need to provide? (This is the pre-class preparation materials)

The principle of backward design is not intuitive for most academic faculty who tend to craft courses in the order that they teach them. However, a TBL course or module will be much easier to create if designed using backward design principles. This section will go through each of these steps one by one, as is illustrated in Fig. 2.1.

2.2 Design Steps

Step 1: Situational Factors
Step 2: Learning Objectives
Step 3: Application Activities
Step 4: Readiness Assurance Activities
Step 5: Preparation/Learning Materials
Step 6: Colleague/Peer Review
Step 7: Piloting

Step 1 Situational Factors	**Consider the Situational Factors** Identify factors that will affect learning.
Step 2 Learning Objectives	**Create Learning Objectives** Decide what you want learners to be able to DO as a result of each TBL module
Step 3 Application Activities	**Create Application Activites** Create applications that are directly aligned to your objectives and meet the requirements of the 4 Ss (Significant Problem, Same Problem, Specific Choice, Simultaneous Report).
Step 4 Readiness Assurance Activities	**Design the Readiness Assurance Process** Write RATs that are foundational to the applications and make sure that they match the TBL objectives
Step 5 Preparation/ Learning Materials	**Identify and/or Develop Preparation Materials** Identify preparation materials that are foundational to RATs. Alternatively, you can create a lecture, online module, or a compilation of different readings that serve as the preparation for the students.
Step 6 Colleague/Peer Review	**Request Colleagues to Review Module** Request colleagues to review entire module: the peer review can take place within a course committee, a TBL curriculum committee, or informally with a colleague.
Step 7 Piloting	**Pilot Module** Pilot your module before it goes "live": if you don't have the opportunity to pilot it, solicit feedback from your students after the TBL session to ascertain their impression of the exercise.

Fig. 2.1 Design steps

2.2.1   Step 1: Situational Factors: Consider the Situational Factors

The success of a TBL course or module frequently hinges on what the learners are required to navigate outside the course. Because so much of TBL requires pre-class preparation, if the learners have a significant workload outside of their TBL class time that interferes with their preparation, it will hinder their ability to come to class prepared. For this reason, examination of the situational factors surrounding the TBL course is essential.

Particularly if a school is planning a curriculum overhaul in which many courses are planning on converting to TBL, it is wise for the course directors to coordinate with each other so as not to overload their students by giving too much reading or too many RATs on the same day.

Clinical course directors need also consider reading burden if their students have overnight call or other situational factors impacting preparation.

In considering your situational factors, think about what your students are required to learn, how much time they have to learn it, what other responsibilities they are managing, and their level of experience and maturity.

> **Example 1**
> You are teaching in a medical school with 120 students. The school teaches in "organ system blocks" so that only one basic science course is taught at a time. All courses are integrated so that pathology, physiology and pharmacology are included in each block.
>
> You decide to transform your second year neuroscience and behavior course to TBL. Situational factors include the following:
>
> - Students are in their second year so they can tolerate some, but not a lot of ambiguity
> - The course is integrated so input from fellow faculty is important when designing objectives, assessments, and activities
> - Since there isn't a concurrent basic science course they can manage a fairly rigorous and challenging pre-class preparation workload

2.2.2   Step 2: Learning Objectives: Create Your Learning Objectives

Create learning objectives based on what you want learners to be able to DO as a result of each module, and make sure the objectives match both your applications and your RATs.

One of the most difficult tasks for faculty is writing objectives. Instructors often want their students to KNOW content, but they have difficulty articulating why they want their students to know this content beyond the fact that IT'S IMPORTANT TO KNOW THIS STUFF.

In order for students to appreciate the relevance of the content you want to relay to them, you must illustrate how it will assist them to be better health care providers. TBL is an excellent strategy to help you demonstrate relevance, because it enables you to craft applications in which students can see themselves using knowledge to solve real life problems.

The objectives you create, however, must be at a higher level than knowledge objectives. If you are utilizing Bloom's taxonomy, aim for objectives in the categories of "Application," "Analysis," Synthesis" or "Evaluation" [2]. Good verbs to use when writing learning objectives include "Choose," "Differentiate," "Propose," "Select" and "Compare." Avoid verbs such as "Understand," "Appreciate," "Define," "Name," "State," "Describe," and "Indicate."

Example 2

For the module defined as "The Neuropsychiatric Manifestations of Alcohol Abuse," in our hypothetical neuroscience course, objectives may include the following:

By the end of this module, the student will:

1. Identify those portions of the brain most sensitive to the impact of alcohol abuse.
2. Compare and contrast the different neuropsychiatric disorders that result from excessive alcohol use.
3. Differentiate between primary mood disorders and alcohol related mood disorders.
4. Diagnose a patient presenting with an alcohol use disorder.
5. Choose the most appropriate treatment for a patient presenting to the physician with an alcohol use disorder.

2.2.3 Step 3: Application Activities: Create Your Application Activities

Your application activities are the most important components of your Team-Based Learning module, so considerable time and effort should be taken to create a good application. Most applications should be case-based and clinically oriented, since most health science students will be entering clinical fields. However, it is appropriate for some cases to be laboratory-based because of the scientific bases of health related fields. In all instances, the applications should be directly aligned to your objectives and should meet the requirements of the 4 Ss (Significant Problem, Same Problem, Specific Choice, Simultaneous Report).

In his chapter "Creating Effective Team Assignments" in *TBL in Health Professions Education* [3], Larry Michaelsen describes the different levels of assignments to promote higher-level learning:

Lowest level: "Make a list"
Example: "List the possible diagnoses that are consistent with the patient data in this case"
Characteristic: Not very challenging, leads to low accountability, doesn't adequately utilize the talent of the team, members are not sufficiently engaged.
Intermediate Level: "Make a choice"
Example: "Which diagnosis (from a list of 5 plausible alternatives) is most likely based on the patient data in this case?"
Characteristic: Engaging, relatively challenging, but still does not draw the most potential from the team.
Highest level: "Make a Specific Choice"
Example: "Which indicator (from a list of five plausible alternatives) is most crucial to making a correct diagnosis in this case?"
Characteristic: Requires high level of cognitive skill, necessitating whole power of the team. Requires learners to make multiple discriminations and perform a sophisticated analysis of content application.

Most instructors new to TBL are accustomed to designing multiple-choice assessment items at the "Make a Choice" level. Therefore, writing applications at the "Make a Specific Choice" level requires some extra effort.

Expending this effort to design high quality applications at the "Make a Specific Choice" level will pay off. When applications reach the "Make a Specific Choice" level, teams engage in high-energy conversations during the "intra-team" (within the team) discussions, they require considerable time to achieve consensus, and they engage in similar high levels of energy and enthusiasm during the "inter- team" (among teams) exchanges following whole class revelation of team choices.

All applications should be tied to their objectives. In Example 3, the application exercise is directly aligned with objectives #3 and #4 articulated in the "Learning Objectives" section of our hypothetical course. Objective #3: differentiate between primary mood disorders and alcohol related mood disorders; Objective #4 diagnose a patient presenting with an alcohol induced neuropsychiatric disorder.

This application is particularly challenging because it requires the students to first consider the most likely diagnoses, and then decide what information is most crucial in order to rule in or rule out their hypothetical diagnoses.

The application requires considerable thought and multiple discriminations. Students will most likely be drawn between answers "B" and "D." The correct answer is "D" (Past psychiatric history focusing on prior mood disorder), because if the patient has a past history of a primary mood disorder, then he is more likely to have a diagnosis of major depression. However if he does not, then the likelihood is that he has a primary diagnosis of an alcohol use disorder. "B" (Further information regarding his substance use: withdrawal? preoccupation? tolerance? etc.) will give more information about the nature of an alcohol related disorder, but only "D" will differentiate between the two syndromes.

Example 3

For the module in our hypothetical neuroscience course, an example of a "Make a *Specific* Choice" applications is as follows: (note: this is a modification of Dwight Wolf's "Substance Abuse" module in the Team-Based Learning Collaborative resource bank, (www.teambasedlearning.org)

"A 27-year-old man presents in your clinic for evaluation. He reports a one-year history of low mood, crying episodes occurring several times per week and profound hopelessness. His appetite has markedly decreased but there has been no weight loss. He no longer enjoys activities and has lost touch with his previous circle of friends. He reported significant concentration difficulties, but nevertheless has managed to continue to perform well in his employment as a computer programmer. He described that his fiancé terminated her relationship with him approximately six months ago and stated, at this point; "I guess I started drinking a little more after that." Despite the stressors, he denies any suicidal ideation. You continue with the history, focusing on potential issues of substance abuse. He reported that he first began drinking during his teenage years, with occasional sips of beer. He stated that he drank more frequently and drank to intoxication on a regular (approximately twice per month) basis while in college. He reported his intake to be no heavier than that of his peers. He reported occasional sporadic drinking following college, but rarely drank to intoxication. He began drinking more heavily concurrent with starting his present job approximately 1½ years ago. He reported using alcohol to "unwind" after work and felt that the alcohol allowed him to relax more in frequent social interactions after work. He had difficulty recalling the progression of his current intake, but stated it started with "about a six-pack" and has progressed to 8-12 beers per day at present.

1. What further information would be **most helpful** in clarifying his diagnosis?

    A. Family history, focusing on substance abuse and mood disorders
    B. Further information regarding his substance use (withdrawal? preoccupation? tolerance? etc.)
    C. Laboratory testing
    D. Past psychiatric history focusing on prior mood disorder
    E. Physical examination"

2.2.4 Step 4: Readiness Assurance Activities: Design Your Readiness Assurance Process

Designing your readiness assurance process is really more than one step, since it involves

- Writing RATs that are foundational to the applications
- Making sure that the RATs match the TBL objectives

When instructors first start creating TBL modules, their instinct is usually to locate an advanced assignment, typically a chapter or article, and then write the RAT to match the assignment. However, it is vital to remember the purpose of the readiness assurance test: that learners have the basic understanding of the principles necessary to do the work of the application activities. Therefore, a good RAT, just like a good application, must be directly tied to the objectives of the module.

One way to map out your readiness assurance test would be review everything your students might need to learn in order to answer the applications you have created and to map out your RAT questions accordingly.

Example 4

Looking back at our neuroscience module, we may need to create RAT questions on:

- diagnostic criteria of alcohol use disorders
- diagnostic criteria of alcohol related mood disorders, including associated signs, symptoms, and laboratory values.
- emergency treatment of alcohol use disorders including alcohol withdrawal
- pharmacology of drugs used to treat alcohol use disorders

Following is a 3-part readiness assurance test question that comes from the same "Substance Abuse" module as our sample application. This 3-part RAT item is straightforward and requires less critical thinking then the application. The assumption is that students who do basic preparation should be able to manage these questions on an individual test. The items here are meant to ensure that students are able to recognize the basic signs and symptoms of alcohol withdrawal, be able to choose the most appropriate management in the emergency setting, and can select the best drug for treatment of alcohol abuse.

Once the students master the basic knowledge and principles of a RAT such as this one, they can then be presented with a complex real world case of an individual with an alcohol use disorder and come up with "specific choice" solutions to more challenging and thought provoking problems.

As you proceed through your applications, you will be able to build a test blueprint of RAT items. It is important to periodically check back with your objectives to make sure that all the RATs basically match up with the objectives, but if you refer back to your applications, and your applications and objectives match, your RATs and objectives should match as well.

Example 5

"A 45-year-old man presents to the emergency room with a sprained ankle sustained in a fall. He reports a 25-year history of daily heavy drinking. His current intake is in excess of one quart of liquor per day, but he reported that he has not had a drink in "a couple of days." He appears emaciated, tremulous, slightly confused and irritable on examination. His vital signs are as follows:

- BP 160/100, pulse 120
- laboratory values: electrolyte panel within normal limits
- liver function tests:

  - SGOT 40 (NR 8-20)
  - SGPT 35 (NR 8-20)
  - Total bilirubin 1.0 (NR 0.1-1.0)

- CBC normal except for mild anemia, with macrocytosis (MCV 120, normal range 76-96 fl.)

1. Which treatment intervention should you administer first in the emergency room?

   a. IV Glucose and thiamine
   b. Naloxone and flumazanil
   c. Naloxone and Vitamin B12
   d. **Thiamine and folate**
   e. Vitamin B12 and folate

2. Which condition poses the greatest immediate risk for this patient?

   a. **Alcohol withdrawal**
   b. Aspiration pneumonia
   c. Cirrhosis
   d. Dementia
   e. Pancreatitis

3. Which drug would be most useful to treat his alcohol craving through its action on the glutamate system?

   a. **acamprosate**
   b. clonidine
   c. disulfiram
   d. naloxone
   e. oxazepam"

2.2.5   Step 5: Preparation/Learning Materials: Identify and/or Develop the Preparation Materials

Most instructors believe they should locate the ideal readings before they write their RATs. However, identifying pre-class preparation materials should not take place before developing your modules. Ideally, you could even write your RAT without even having any preparation materials identified. If your items are appropriately case-based (in the USMLE-United States Medical Licensing Examination format) and not tricky or factoid, they could be supported by a variety of preparatory materials. The advantage of writing your RAT items first and identifying pre-class preparation materials afterwards is that you will be less likely to be tempted to choose picky and fact-based questions that are grounded in the reading material.

Furthermore, you will find it easier to update your readings without having to significantly change your RATs as your course changes over time.

Only after putting together your objectives and your applications should you begin to locate or develop your pre-class preparation materials. Identifying appropriate materials for pre-class preparation can often be quite challenging, since succinct reading to support RATs (especially in the basic sciences) is often not readily available. For example, in the neurosciences, textbooks have expanded to epic proportions. Students often joke about how they can be used as excellent doorstops or weights for bodybuilding.

Many TBL instructors create learning guides to serve as preparation materials that are foundational to RATs. Alternatively, one can create a lecture, online module, or a compilation of different readings that serve as the preparation for the students.

Most important is that you assign specific and appropriate preparatory materials for your students. If you assign suggested reading or reading that is too long or difficult, your TBL exercises will be compromised before you even get started. In general, a reasonable assignment for a basic science course might include approximately six hours of out-of-class preparation for a two hours in-class TBL exercise.

Example 6

For our "theoretical" neuroscience course, pre-class preparation might be the following:

- 1 chapter on alcohol use disorders
- 1 chapter on mood disorders
- 1 online module on addiction, dependence and withdrawal including drugs used to treat alcohol use disorders
- 1 laboratory session examining brains affected by dementia including alcohol related dementia

2.2.6 Step 6: Colleague/Peer Review: Request One or More Colleagues to Review Your TBL Module

After you develop a first draft of your TBL module, sharing materials with peers can be very helpful in improving the overall product. Peer review can take place within a course committee, a TBL curriculum committee or informally with a colleague. In the event that you are developing your modules in isolation, finding a consultant to help you review it through the Team-Based Learning Collaborative is another option. www.teambasedlearning.org

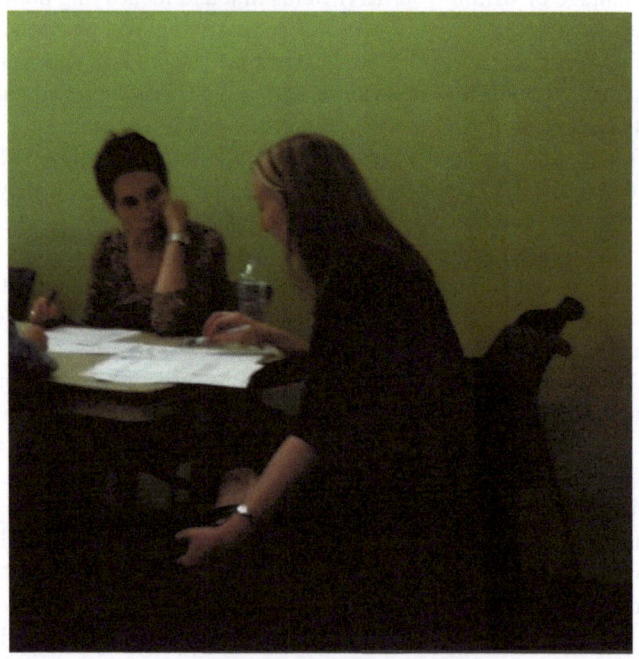

Peer-review can reveal unseen flaws in every component of the module. It is necessary no matter how long one has been developing TBL materials. Both the content of the material covered and the structure of the RATs and applications can be interpreted differently when seen by "fresh" eyes.

2.2.7   Step 7: Piloting: Pilot Your TBL Module Before It Goes Live

One can never predict how a module will perform until it is actually presented to a group of learners. Piloting your TBL module with students will give you the opportunity to obtain valuable feedback so you can make modifications before adopting it into your course.

If your course takes place only once a year, you may not have the opportunity to pilot your module with the same kinds of students as the ones you will be teaching in your TBL course. In such an instance, try using learners from another class (such as 3rd or 4th year students for a 2nd year course).

If you don't have the opportunity to pilot your module, solicit feedback from your students after the TBL session to ascertain their impression of the exercise. Ask what they feel they learned from the class, and make note of whether your objectives were met.

2.3   Implementation Steps

The following section will review some of the practical issues involved in setting up your TBL course, as is illustrated in Fig. 2.2:

1. Team Formation
2. Orientation
3. Incentive structure
4. Appeals
5. Student Peer Assessment/Evaluation

2.3.1   Step 1: Team Formation

One of the most important decisions a course instructor makes is the strategy for forming student teams. Important principles that should be considered include the following:

- Faculty must form the teams. Students should NEVER be allowed to form their own teams. Student-formed teams tend to be homogenous and unequal, and will lead to dysfunctional behavior in the long run.
- Whatever quality will serve as an advantage for the teams should be distributed as equally as possible. For example, if clinical experience might be an advantage, attempt to distribute students who have clinical experience equally.

Step 1 Team Formation	**Form Teams** Form heterogeneous teams that include 5 to 7 members. Keep teams together for at least the duration of the course, preferably for an entire semester/year. Ensure that the team formation process is transparent. Do not allow students to self-select teams.
Step 2 Orientation	**Orient Students** Perform an orientation using TBL methodology in which the pre-class preparation is either a handout about TBL or materials about the course such as a course syllabus. Orientation is also a good time to transparently form the teams.
Step 3 Incentive Structure	**Create Incentive Structure** Ensure that both individual and group accountability is in place for optimal team functioning: a significant portion of the grade must come from both individual and team efforts.
Step 4 Appeals	**Provide Opportunity for Appeals** Allow teams to have the opportunity to appeal an item in writing: either by explaining why their choice is the correct answer, or by re-writing a poorly constructed item. Students should construct their appeal as a team, ideally during class time to ensure that the appeals process is a team effort and not conducted by an individual member.
Step 5 Student Peer Assessment / Evaluation	**Conduct Student Peer Assessment/Evaluation** Conduct peer evaluation to provide valuable feedback to the students in terms of their interpersonal and communication skills. This is a core component of accountability in TBL, preventing the "social loafing" which can erode small group effectiveness.

Fig. 2.2 Implementation steps

- In the long run, heterogeneous teams are far preferable to homogenous teams [4]. Attempt to avoid teams that are too similar. Try to avoid, for example, teams that are all one gender.
- Aim for teams that include 5–7 students in number. Teams of less than five will lack the talent for challenging problems. Teams greater than seven will find it difficult to become cohesive and may form into "sub-teams."
- Whenever possible, be transparent when forming teams. Transparency can be accomplished by lining up students and having them count according to the number of teams you need. Try to avoid a system in which students are stratified by grades or another system in which you have to be secretive regarding the team formation system.
- Once your teams are formed, keep them together for at least the duration of the course, preferably for a whole semester or year.
- If you anticipate that you will have learners that will be out for many of your sessions (such as postgraduate residents), make sure you have large enough teams at the beginning of your course to compensate for absences in subsequent sessions.

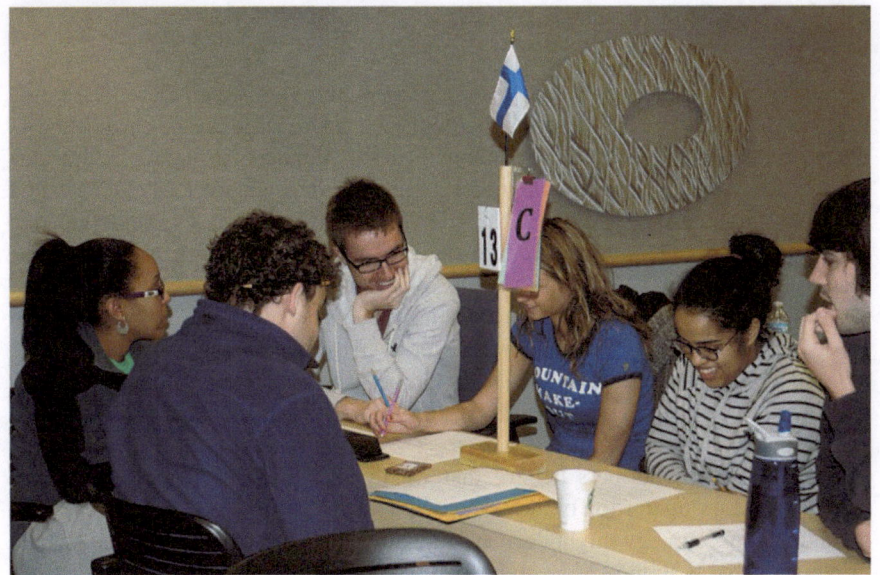

2.3.2   Step 2: Orientation

All learners benefit from course orientation, but students who are novices to Team-Based Learning will derive particular benefit. If you are introducing TBL into your curriculum and plan on using the method for several courses, schedule a full course session to introduce your students just to the didactic method itself. A "mini-TBL 101" session can be utilized in which you enable your students to experience TBL in a non-threatening and fun way.

Orientation sessions can be particularly useful for educating students about some of the more controversial aspects of the method such as group grades and peer evaluation. Students quickly discover during orientation that a team can perform better than an individual and the experience helps them better accept and appreciate the rules of individual and group accountability.

Some instructors will perform an orientation using the TBL methodology in which the pre-class preparation is either a handout about Team-Based Learning or materials about the course such as a course syllabus. Orientation is also a good time to transparently put together the teams that will last for the rest of the course block or semester.

Even if your students are familiar with TBL, a brief orientation is important at the start of every course to help the students become familiar with the particulars of YOUR course. Use this orientation to get your student teams working together for the first time so the process of "team norming" can begin in a non-threatening environment before grading begins. Many TBL instructors will determine the particular grade weights (percentage of grades assigned to individual, group and peer evaluation) during orientation [5].

2.3.3   Step 3: Incentive Structure

The principle of individual and group accountability in Team-Based Learning requires that in every TBL course a particular incentive structure be established so that students are held responsible for both their individual and group work. Students are incentivized, usually through grades, to prepare for their work as evidenced by their performance on the IRATs, the GRATs, and in some cases the application activities. It is also recommended that students conduct peer evaluations, both formative and summative, as another means of accountability.

Although no consensus exists regarding the exact percentage of the students' grade that should come from individual work versus group work, the primary principle in TBL is that each component should be weighed so that students are motivated to prepare for their individual tests, as well as motivated to participate and do well in the group process.

Many TBL practitioners believe that weighing a greater proportion of grade weight on the group portion of the grade will improve group process, but some have argued that this strategy might decrease individual accountability. The fundamental principle is that both individual and group accountability must be in place for optimal team functioning. Therefore, a significant portion of the grade must come from both individual and team efforts.

Many advocate asking the students during orientation to decide upon the details of the incentive structure; e.g. the percentage of the grade that will go to individual work, group work, and peer evaluation. Including students on the details of the incentive structure, with guidelines such as a range for each component (e.g. individual work can count 30–70%, group work can count 30–70%, peer evaluation can count 5–10%) helps create "buy-in" for the course. Generally, students choose the highest possible percentages for group work once they discover that the team always scores higher than the individual.

2.3.4   Step 4: Appeals

Although the appeals process is relatively brief, occurring between readiness assurance and application activities, it is an essential component of TBL and should not be discounted. The primary purpose of the appeals process is to incentivize teams to review the material that they missed. Ideally, the review should occur as quickly as possible after the GRAT, so that the teams can obtain immediate feedback (the most effective kind) on the items that were confusing to them.

If the teams discover that a particular item is coded incorrectly, they then have the opportunity to appeal that item in writing to the instructor. They can also rewrite a poorly constructed item. They should construct their appeal as a team, ideally during class time to ensure that the appeals process is a team effort and not conducted by an individual member.

Time constraints will sometimes force instructors to move the appeals process to outside of class time. Taking appeals outside of class time can be a risk, since the appeals process lends itself to individual rather than team effort.

Allowing students a brief period of time to work on appeals will not only prevent the phenomenon of individuals creating multiple team appeals, it will also significantly improve the facilitator feedback portion of readiness assurance. Teams will have the opportunity to clarify misunderstandings of simple concepts on their own, enabling discussing of more complex subjects.

2.3.5 Step 5: Student Peer Assessment/Evaluation

A core component of accountability in Team-Based Learning is peer assessment or evaluation. When conducted appropriately, peer evaluation can provide valuable feedback to the students in terms of their interpersonal and communication skills, while at the same time preventing the "social loafing" which can erode small group effectiveness. A variety of different methods of peer assessment exist, which are described in detail in other texts [3]. Some of the basic principles when administering peer evaluation include the following:

- Peer evaluation is the most culturally sensitive component of TBL, so what works in one setting may not work in another. For example, Michaelsen found that business students are quite accepting of discriminating quantitative peer evaluations in which one student is required to be graded higher than another. In contrast, medical students are hostile to this method, and much more comfortable with a system in which all peers could be given equal credit [6].
- Peer evaluation is not intuitive, and students need to be taught how to do it. Indeed, a separate orientation on peer evaluation alone can be very helpful to instruct on the method and ease anxiety [7].
- Both formative and summative evaluations should take place. Formative evaluation is useful not only for the student receiving feedback but also for the evaluator to learn how to perform the method.
- Both quantitative and qualitative evaluations are useful. Quantitative evaluation gives the method "teeth" so that it makes a difference in terms of accountability. Qualitative feedback is essential for helping the students obtain the feedback they need to be better team players.
- Peer evaluations should not be administered too often. A midterm formative evaluation and an end of term summative evaluation are standard for a course of six weeks or longer. For very brief courses, qualitative non-graded evaluation may be appropriate. Asking students to perform peer feedback often or before they have had sufficient time to "norm" as a team can interfere with group cohesion and be counterproductive.

References

1. Wiggins G, McTighe J. Understanding by design (Merrill Education/ASCD College Textbook Series); 1998
2. Bloom BS, Hastings JT, Madaus G. Taxonomy of educational objectives, handbook 1: cognitive domain. New York: McKay; 1956.
3. Michaelsen LK, Parmelee DX, McMahon KK, Levine RE. Team-Based Learning for Health Professions Education: A Guide to Using Small Groups for Improving Learning. Chapter 2. Sterling, VA: Stylus; 2008.
4. Michaelsen LK. Three Keys to Using Learning Groups Effectively. Adapted from the Professional and Organizational Development Network Essay Series Teaching Excellence: Toward the Best in the Academy, vol. 9. Ames, IA: POD Network; 1997–1998.
5. Michaelsen LK, Sweet M, Parmelee DX, eds. Team-Based Learning: Small Group Learning's Next Big Step. San Francisco, New Directions in Teaching and Learning, Number116 California: Jossey-Bass; 2008.
6. Levine RE, Kelly PA, Karakoc T, Haidet P. Peer evaluation in a clinical clerkship: students' attitudes, experiences, and correlations with traditional assessments. Acad Psychiatry. 2007;31(1):19–24.
7. Michaelsen LK, Schultheiss EE. Making feedback helpful. Organ Behav Teach Rev. 1988;13(1):109–13.

Chapter 3
What Factors Will Facilitate or Sabotage my Success?

Team-Based Learning is an exciting new instructional modality, yet not every school or faculty member who has introduced TBL has been successful in maintaining long-term implementation. Evaluation of dissemination attempts [1] have revealed that certain aspects of TBL implementation can have great impact on the success of a TBL course or curriculum.

Once your module is developed, a variety of factors can make or break the TBL experience:

- Buy-in
- Organization and Coordination
- The Right Room
- Facilitator vs. Lecturer
- Too Much Too Often
- Poor Incentive Structure
- Poor Exercises

3.1 Buy-In

The more faculty, students, and administrators you have on board when you decide to introduce your TBL course, the higher the likelihood you will be successful in your implementation. Any stakeholders in the course or curriculum should be educated regarding the reason for the course revision, the advantages of TBL over conventional didactic methods, and the amount of time and effort required to convert from previous traditional courses to TBL courses.

Stakeholders who do not understand TBL can serve as active or passive saboteurs of the new method. Students may prove hostile when confronted with copious

R. E. Levine, P. D. Hudes, *How-to Guide for Team-Based Learning*, IAMSE Manuals, https://doi.org/10.1007/978-3-030-62923-6_3

amounts of pre-class preparation, in-class tests, and the requirement to work in teams when they have not had previous positive experiences with small group work.

Faculty forced to adopt a new method of teaching because of top-down change can rebel against the effort required to learn the method and develop new teaching materials.

Administrators focused on student evaluations may not appreciate that TBL can generate increases in student engagement and performance while at the same time making a small but vocal minority of students unhappy about having to do more work.

"Buy in" is one of the reasons for developing a comprehensive orientation for faculty, staff, and students prior to beginning your TBL course.

3.2   Organization and Coordination

Even when faculty are knowledgeable and enthusiastic about implementing TBL, a curriculum implementation can be damaged if it is not conducted in a coordinated and organized fashion. For example, if a biochemistry course, an anatomy course, and a physiology course, which run concurrently all decide to convert to TBL simultaneously, and the course directors don't meet and share information about quantity of pre-class preparatory materials and timing of RATs, the students could be overwhelmed with out of class work.

Students will become frustrated having 3 RATs in 3 different courses on the same day. While this example is extreme, even modest implementations have better chances of success when faculty and staff coordinate with each other so that student workload can be managed and testing does not become onerous.

3.3   The Right Room

TBL can be done in almost any room large enough to accommodate a class. Nevertheless, certain types of classrooms are better than others for TBL to take place. The best type of classroom is a flat one in which students can sit close to each other around small tables so that everyone can see and speak to each other easily for small group work.

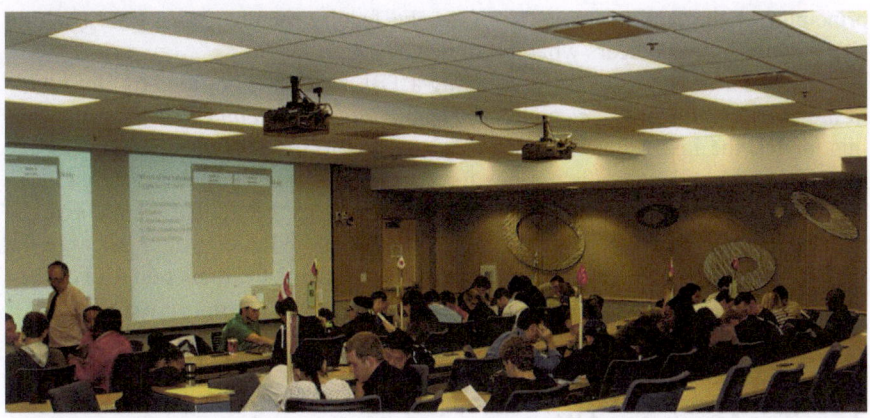

Faculty should be careful to avoid using large round tables that inhibit speech across the table—a small rectangular or oval table is better so that all students can easily interact with other students in their team. For "inter-group" interaction students should be able to easily see all of the other students in the room, and if possible, microphones should be present so everyone can hear.

The worst type of classrooms are those in which students are forced to be in steep amphitheatre type rooms with fixed chairs that cannot swivel around for them to see each other easily. These types of classrooms not only interfere with team dynamics but they also promote lecturing over facilitating.

3.4   Facilitator vs. Lecturer

A significant challenge for faculty new to TBL is transitioning from lecturer to facilitator. Facilitating a TBL classroom can initially be daunting—the classroom is often loud—students can seem unruly and argumentative, and the comfortable rhythm associated with a lecture is no longer present. Moreover—instructors who are accustomed to delivering content must now hold back what they know until they can draw out from the students their thoughts and questions.

For many faculty, it is far easier to answer questions than serve as a facilitator of discussion between the teams—but as soon as a faculty member starts lecturing, the students very quickly fall silent to listen to the expert.

It is important to appreciate that the students are often better teachers than the faculty. Because students are closer to each other in terms of knowledge and skills, they understand better what their classmates don't know, and therefore they are better at filling in the knowledge gaps and explaining crucial points.

Only by listening to students attempting to explain issues can the faculty understand if the students get it or not. Only by having one team explain an answer to another team can a faculty member appreciate if the teams really understand the principles of the applications. Therefore, the faculty member must hold back on lecturing until he/she hears what the students have to say.

A good format to use while facilitating a TBL session is outlined by Jim Sibley in the book *Team Based Learning for The Social Sciences and Humanities* [2]. In this model, the instructor introduces the students to the session by clarifying the objectives and reviewing the reasons for the lesson. After facilitating the readiness assurance and application activities, the instructor helps the students summarize the main discussion points by asking a question such as "What do you think were the most important principles you learned today?" Reviewing the main points of discussion helps students recognize what they have achieved as a result of the lesson.

3.5 Too Much Too Often

As mentioned earlier, faculty need to be careful when starting a TBL program to not "overload" students with too many RATs. Often new faculty are impressed with the increased engagement that accompanies the readiness assurance process and they mistakenly believe that RATs are the cornerstones of TBL. Students can quickly become disenchanted with a TBL course that burdens them with excessive testing, even one in which otherwise excellent teaching takes place. Only a sampling of preparatory material needs to be tested to assure that the students are ready for the application portion—the "meat" of TBL. A RAT session is not necessary for every application exercise session. Many faculty will conduct an hour of readiness assurance followed by one to three hours of applications.

Peer evaluation is another component of TBL that can be harmful when administered too often. One formative and one summative peer evaluation per course or semester is generally sufficient. Conducting peer evaluations with short courses or giving students frequent peer evaluations can interfere with team cohesion.

3.6 Poor Incentive Structure

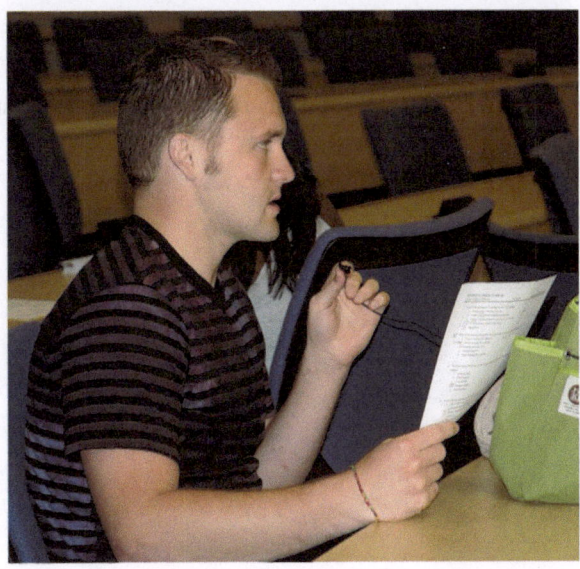

Individual and team accountability are both vital components of the TBL incentive structure. When a course director lacks the ability to incentivize students for both individual and team efforts, the course will suffer significantly. If, for example, a school has a rule that students cannot be graded for large group classes so that coming to TBL is an optional activity, there will be no reason for students to do the pre-class work and students will not be prepared for the readiness assurance or application activities. Not all the students may show up for class (as is the case in many lecture classes) and teams will be underpowered.

If students are only incentivized for individual work then engagement and enthusiasm may diminish during group activities and quieter students will not be encouraged by their teammates to speak. Conversely, an incentive structure in which only team grades are counted may encourage social loafing.

3.7 Poor Exercises

Ultimately, the most important components of your TBL course are your application exercises. The quality of your course will hinge on the quality of these exercises. If the exercises are well designed, in the "make a specific choice" category, and aligned with higher level learning goals, your course will have the best chance of success. Conversely, poorly designed applications, which are not well aligned with learning goals, can lead to low levels of learner engagement and overall dissatisfaction with the course.

References

1. Thompson BM, Schneider VF, Haidet P, Perkowski LC, Richards BF. Factors influencing implementation of team-based learning in health sciences education. Acad Med. 2007a;82(10 Suppl):S53–6.
2. Sweet M, Michaelsen L, eds. Team-based learning in the social sciences and humanities group work that works to generate critical thinking and engagement stylus; 2012.

Chapter 4
How Can I Learn the Knowledge and Skills to get Started?

A variety of resources, groups and meetings exist to help faculty who wish to learn more about teaching with the TBL method. Common strategies for learning TBL teaching skills including the following:

- Reviewing the TBL Collaborative and other websites
- Reading Books and Guides
- Participating in Regional and National Workshops
- Joining the TBL Listserv
- Becoming a TBL Collaborative Member
- Visiting a School
- Inviting a TBL consultant

4.1 Reviewing the TBL Collaborative and Other Websites

These websites provide excellent resources for the implementation of effective TBL:

- Team-Based Learning Collaborative: www.teambasedlearning.org
- IF-AT (Immediate Feedback Assessment Technique): www.epsteineducation.com
- MedEdPORTAL: www.mededportal.org
- National Board of Medical Examiners (NBME) Constructing Written Test Questions for the Basic and Clinical Sciences: www.nbme.org/publications/item-writing-manual.html

4.1.1   Team-Based Learning Collaborative

www.teambasedlearning.org
The mission of the Team-Based Learning Collaborative (TBLC) is to promote the understanding and evolution of Team-Based Learning across the educational community. The purpose of the TBLC is to encourage communication, mutual support and continuing professional development among educators in academia and industry using Team-Based Learning. Through their website, the TBLC hopes to provide a resource of expertise in Team-Based Learning. The website includes information on "getting started," "forming teams," "orienting students," "setting grade weights," "helping students prepare," "the RAP process," "application exercises," "facilitation skills," and "peer evaluation."

4.1.2   IF-AT (Immediate Feedback Assessment Technique)

www.epsteineducation.com
The Immediate Feedback Assessment Technique, also known as the IF-AT, is used for the Group Readiness Assurance Test to provide students a means of obtaining immediate feedback on their answers.

The IF-AT is a multiple-choice answer form with a thin opaque film covering the answer options. Instead of using a pencil to fill in a circle, students scratch off their answer as if scratching a lottery ticket. If the answer is correct, a star appears somewhere within the rectangle.

4.1.3   MedEdPORTAL

www.mededportal.org
MedEdPORTAL is a open access journal for medical and oral health teaching materials, assessment tools, and faculty development resources. A growing number of TBL resources is available to health science faculty through the MedEdPORTAL website.

4.1.4   National Board of Medical Examiners (NBME) Constructing Written Test Questions for the Basic and Clinical Sciences

www.nbme.org/publications/item-writing-manual.html
Writing high quality multiple choice questions is essential for the success of your readiness assurance process. This manual was written to help faculty improve the quality of the multiple-choice questions written for their examinations. It provides an overview of item formats, concentrating on the traditional one-best-answer and matching formats. It reviews issues related to technical item flaws and issues related to item content. The manual also provides basic information to help faculty review statistical indices of item quality after test administration. The examples focus on undergraduate medical education, though the general approach to item writing may be useful for assessing examinees at other levels.

4.2   Reading Books or Guides

4.2.1   Books

Four books have been written specifically about Team-Based Learning:

1. **Team-Based Learning: A Transformative Use of Small Groups in College Teaching**
   Michaelsen LK, Knight AB, Fink LD, eds., Sterling, VA: Stylus; 2004.
   This was the first book published about TBL. It offers a general overview and would be useful in any setting. Part I covers the basics (merits and limitations of small groups and teams: the processes for transforming small groups into cohesive teams and for creating effective assignments). In Part II, teachers from various disciplines describe their use of TBL. Part III offers a synopsis of the major lessons to be learned from the experiences of the teachers who have used TBL. The appendices answer frequently asked questions, include useful forms and exercises, and offer advice on peer evaluations and grading.
2. **Team-Based Learning for Health Professions Education: A Guide to Using Small Groups for Improving Learning**
   Michaelsen LK, Parmelee DX, McMahon KK, Levine RE., Sterling, Va: Stylus; 2008.
   This book is an introduction to TBL for health profession educators. It outlines the theory, structure, and process of TBL. It includes chapters in which instructors describe how they apply TBL in their courses with examples that range across undergraduate science courses, basic and clinical sciences courses in medical, sports medicine and nursing education, residencies, and graduate nursing programs. The book concludes with a review and critique of the current scholarship on TBL in the health professions, and charts the needs for future research.

3. **Team-Based Learning: Small Group Learning's Next Big Step**
   Michaelsen LK, Sweet M, Parmelee DX, eds., San Francisco, New Directions in Teaching and Learning, Number 116 Calif: Jossey-Bass; 2008.
   This book is available as paperback and eBook (http://onlinelibrary.wiley.com/doi/ 10.1002/ tl.v2008:116/issuetoc). It describes the practical elements of TBL, how it works in the classroom, and the lessons learned as TBL grows into an interdisciplinary and international practice. Several articles in this volume illustrate the TBL emphasis on learning (versus teaching) by using TBL students' own words to reinforce key ideas. It also includes a chapter that introduces the use of TBL in asynchronous online settings.
4. **Team-Based Learning in the Social Sciences and Humanities Group Work that Works to Generate Critical Thinking and Engagement**
   Sweet M, Michaelsen L, eds., Stylus; 2012.
   The most recent TBL book published (2012), it is available as both a paperback and an eBook. It introduces the elements of TBL and how to apply them in the social sciences and humanities. It describes the four essential elements of TBL—readiness assurance, design of application exercises, permanent teams, peer evaluation—and pays particular attention to the specification of learning outcomes, which can be a unique challenge in these fields. The core of the book consists of examples of how TBL has been incorporated into the cultures of various disciplines. The authors explain why they felt a need to change how they taught and why they chose TBL. Furthermore, each chapter provides examples of the assignments and exercises they use to help their students achieve the specific learning outcomes of their courses.

4.2.2   Guides

These guides offer step-by-step advice on how to implement Team-Based Learning:

1. **A Practical Guide for Medical Teachers**
   Dent J, Harden R eds., Elsevier, 2013, 4th edition. TBL chapter authors: Parmelee D, Hudes P, Michaelsen L.
   This guide is available in paperback and eBook formats. As in its previous editions, it presents and discusses contemporary educational principles, including a chapter about TBL, providing practical help in the delivery of the variety of teaching situations which characterize present-day curricula. Key concepts and tips are presented in a way which indicates both their immediate relevance and practical implications. The topics are presented in a concise format, providing practical tips, answering questions, and giving back-up advice.
2. **Team-Based Learning: A Practical Guide**
   Parmelee D, Michaelsen L, Cook S, Hudes P, AMEE Guide No. 65, 2012. Med Teach. 2012;34(5):e275-87. Epub 2012 Apr 4.

This guide's purpose is to clarify what TBL is and is not, when and how it should be used, and which of its components must be done (and how) for the greatest likelihood of success. The guide also entices those who are still lecturing to consider engaging students into solving real- world clinical practice problems and challenge those using problem-based learning (PBL) or other small group learning activities to add TBL to their teaching repertoire.

4.3   Participating in Regional and National Workshops

As the popularity of TBL has grown, the prevalence of TBL workshops at education meetings has also increased:

- **Team-Based Learning Collaborative (TBLC) Annual Meeting**
  Every year the TBLC www.teambasedlearning.org offers three tracks at its annual meeting: a fundamentals track, an innovation track, and a research track. Novices to TBL can come to the meeting and participate in the "fundamentals track" starting with a pre-meeting "Introduction to TBL" workshop and continuing with workshops in "designing modules," "facilitating skills," "peer evaluation," and other basic skills necessary to implementing a TBL course or module. Participating in the "fundamentals track" is likely one of the best strategies for learning the knowledge and skills to implement TBL.
- **International Association of Medical Science Educators (IAMSE) Annual Meeting**
  At every IAMSE www.iamse.org meeting there are both introductory and advanced workshops in TBL, as well as scholarship generated by TBL practitioners presented during the poster sessions.
- **Association of American Colleges (AAMC) and Group on Educational Affairs (GEA) Meetings**
  There are also frequently TBL workshops presented during regional GEA www.aamc.org/members/gea meetings as well as the Annual meeting of the AAMC www.aamc.org.

4.4   Joining the TBL Listserv

The TBL Listserv www.teambasedlearning.org is an open access service for anyone who wishes to pose questions about Team-Based learning. It is an active list serve and is frequently used by faculty addressing specific problems or looking for other faculty in their specialties.

4.5   Becoming a TBL Collaborative Member

Both institutional and individual memberships in the TBL Collaborative are available through the website www.teambasedlearning.org. Members of the TBLC have access to a large membership directory and are able to obtain contact information of individual members. Faculty can benefit from the expertise of colleagues in different institutions who have been teaching with the TBL method for a longer period of time. TBLC members also have access to a members-only resource bank, workshop materials, the TBL listserv search archive and "Scholarship of Teaching and Learning" resources. Members also receive discounts on TBLC annual meeting conference registration and other TBL materials.

4.6   Visiting a School

Many faculty have found it useful to visit schools in which TBL is the primary instructional strategy. Visiting a real TBL classroom can enable novice faculty to visualize for themselves some of the intangible aspects of organizing and facilitating a TBL class, which are not always explained in conventional workshops. When you visit a TBL school, you can see practical ways to arrange classrooms, organize materials, and manage a large number of real student teams.

4.7   Inviting a TBL Consultant

If an institution is planning on implementing TBL with many or most of its courses, inviting a TBL "expert" can be the most efficient strategy for helping a significant number of course faculty learn the knowledge and skills to become proficient in developing a TBL curriculum. A TBL consultant can come in for anywhere from one to three days and provide fundamental workshops in TBL. Often it is useful to have one consultant visit for one day and then have another consultant return in several months after faculty develop some experience with working on the method and have educated questions about implementation strategies. It is most useful to develop an ongoing relationship with the consultant after the initial contact so that assistance can be provided with continuing questions and review of materials.

References

1. Haidet P, O'Malley KJ, Richards B. An initial experience with "team learning" in medical education. Acad Med. 2002;77:40–4.
2. Searle NS, Haidet P, Kelly PA, Schneider VF, Seidel CL, Richards BF. Team learning in medical education: experiences at ten institutions. Acad Med. 2003;78(10 suppl):S55–8.
3. Levine RE, O'Boyle M, Haidet P, Lynn DJ, Stone MM, Wolf DV, Paniagua FA. Transforming a clinical clerkship with team learning. Teach Learn Med. 2004;16:270–5.
4. Chung EK, Rhee JA, Baik YH, Oh-Sun A. The effect of team-based learning in medical ethics education. Med Teach. 2009;31:1013–7.
5. Koles P, Stolfi A, Borges N, Nelson S, Parmelee D. The impact of team-based learning on medical students' academic performance. Acad Med. 2010;85(11):1739–45.
6. Michaelsen LK, Parmelee DX, McMahon KK, Levine RE. Team-Based Learning for Health Professions Education: A Guide to Using Small Groups for Improving Learning. Chapter 2. Sterling, VA: Stylus; 2008.
7. Wiggins G, McTighe J. Understanding by design (Merrill Education/ASCD College Textbook Series); 1998
8. Bloom BS, Hastings JT, Madaus G. Taxonomy of educational objectives, handbook 1: cognitive domain. New York: McKay; 1956.
9. Michaelsen LK. Three Keys to Using Learning Groups Effectively. Adapted from the Professional and Organizational Development Network Essay Series Teaching Excellence: Toward the Best in the Academy, vol. 9. Ames, IA: POD Network; 1997–1998.
10. Michaelsen LK, Sweet M, Parmelee DX, eds. Team-Based Learning: Small Group Learning's Next Big Step. San Francisco, New Directions in Teaching and Learning, Number116 California: Jossey-Bass; 2008.
11. Levine RE, Kelly PA, Karakoc T, Haidet P. Peer evaluation in a clinical clerkship: students' attitudes, experiences, and correlations with traditional assessments. Acad Psychiatry. 2007;31(1):19–24.
12. Michaelsen LK, Schultheiss EE. Making feedback helpful. Organ Behav Teach Rev. 1988;13(1):109–13.
13. Thompson BM, Schneider VF, Haidet P, Perkowski LC, Richards BF. Factors influencing implementation of team-based learning in health sciences education. Acad Med. 2007a;82(10 Suppl):S53–6.
14. Sweet M, Michaelsen L, eds. Team-based learning in the social sciences and humanities group work that works to generate critical thinking and engagement stylus; 2012.

Bibliography

Abdelkhalek N, Hussein A, Gibbs T, Hamdy H. Using team-based learning to prepare medical students for future problem-based learning. Med Teach. 2010;32:123–9.

Beatty SJ, Kelley KA, Metzger AH, Bellebaum KL, McAuley JW. Team-based learning in therapeutics workshop sessions. Am J Pharm Educ. 2009;73:100.

Bloom BS, Hastings JT, Madaus G. Taxonomy of educational objectives, handbook 1: cognitive Domain. New York: McKay; 1956.

Chung EK, Rhee JA, Baik YH, OS A. The effect of team-based learning in medical ethics education. Med Teach. 2009;31:1013–7.

Clark MC, Nguyen HT, Bray C, Levine RE. Team-based learning in an undergraduate nursing course. J Nurs Educ. 2008;47:111–7.

Conway SE, Johnson JL, Ripley TL. Integration of team-based learning strategies into a cardiovascular module. Am J Pharm Educ. 2010;74:35.

Dunaway GA. Adaption of team learning to an introductory graduate pharmacology course. Teach Learn Med. 2005;17:56–62.

Fink LD. Creating significant learning experiences: an integrated approach to designing college courses (Jossey-Bass Higher and Adult Education). 2003.

Gladwell M. The tipping point: how little things can make a big difference. Boston, MA: Little, Brown, and Company; 2000.

Haidet P, Clark MB, Frazer C, Yang C, Breault C, Cherry R. An interprofessional curriculum in quality improvement for medical and nursing students. Paper presented at: 33rd Annual Meeting of the Society of General Internal Medicine; April 29, 2010; Minneapolis, Minnesota.

Haidet P, Fecile ML. Team-based learning: a promising strategy to foster active learning in cancer education. J Cancer Educ. 2006;21:125–8.

Haidet P, Levine R, Parmelee D, Crow S, Kennedy F, Kelly A, Perkowski L, Michaelsen L, Richards B. Perspective: guidelines for reporting team-based learning activities in the medical and health sciences education literature. Acad Med. 2012;87(3):292–9.

Haidet P, Morgan RO, O'Malley K, Moran BJ, Richards BF. A controlled trial of active versus passive learning strategies in a large group setting. Adv Health Sci Educ. 2004;9:15–27.

Haidet P, O'Malley KJ, Richards B. An initial experience with "team learning" in medical education. Acad Med. 2002;77:40–4.

Hunt DP, Haidet P, Coverdale JH, Richards B. The effect of using team learning in an evidence-based medicine course for medical students. Teach Learn Med. 2003;15:131–9.

Interprofessional Education Collaborative Expert Panel. Core competencies for interprofessional collaborative practice: report of an expert panel. Washington. In: DC; 2011.

Johnson DW, Johnson RT, Smith KA. Constructive controversy. Change. 2000;32:29–37.

Ju YS. Evaluation of a team-based learning tutor training workshop on research and publication ethics by faculty and staff participants. J Educ Eval Health Prof. 2009;6:5.

Keeher J. Collaborative learning: a sourcebook for higher education, vol. 2. National Center for Teaching, Learning, and Assessment: State College, PA; 1994.

Kelly PA, Haidet P, Schneider V, Searle N, Seidel CL, Richards BF. A comparison of in class learner engagement across lecture, problem-based learning, and team learning using the STROBE classroom observation tool. Teach Learn Med. 2005;17:112–8.

Kim SY. Students' evaluation of a team-based course on research and publication ethics: attitude change in medical school graduate students. J Educ Eval Health Prof. 2008;5:3. https://doi.org/10.3352/jeehp.2008.5.3.

Koles P, Nelson S, Stolfi A, Parmelee D, Destephen D. Active learning in a year 2 pathology curriculum. Med Educ. 2005;39:1045–55.

Koles P, Stolfi A, Borges N, Nelson S, Parmelee D. The impact of team-based learning on medical students' academic performance. Acad Med. 2010;85(11):1739–45.

Kuhne-Eversmann L, Eversmann T, Fischer MR. Team- and case-based learning to activate participants and enhance knowledge: an evaluation of seminars in Germany. J Contin Educ Health Prof. 2008;28:165–71.

Letassy NA, Fugate SE, Medina MS, Stroup JS, Britton ML. Using team-based learning in an endocrine module taught across two campuses. Am J Pharm Educ. 2008;72:103.

Levine RE, Kelly PA, Karakoc T, Haidet P. Peer evaluation in a clinical clerkship: students' attitudes, experiences, and correlations with traditional assessments. Acad Psychiatry. 2007;31(1):19–24.

Levine RE, O'Boyle M, Haidet P, Lynn DJ, Stone MM, Wolf DV, Paniagua FA. Transforming a clinical clerkship with team learning. Teach Learn Med. 2004;16:270–5.

Liaison Committee on Medical Education. Accreditation Standards (www.lcme.org/ standard. htm). Accessed July 19, 2011.

Liaison Committee on Medical Education. Functions and Structure of a Medical School. http://www.lcme.org/functions2011may.pdf. Accessed November 17, 2011.

McInerney MJ. Team-based learning enhances long-term retention and critical thinking in an undergraduate microbial physiology course. Microbiol Educ J. 2003;4:3–12.

McMahon KK. Team-based learning. In: Jeffries WB, Huggett KN, editors. An introduction to medical teaching. Dordrecht, The Netherlands: Springer; 2010.

MedEdPORTAL. www.aamc.org/mededportal Accessed November 17, 2011.

Mennenga HA, Smyer T. A model for easily incorporating team-based learning into nursing education. Int J Nurs Educ Scholarsh. 2010;7:article 4.

Michaelsen LK. Three Keys to Using Learning Groups Effectively. Adapted from the Professional and Organizational Development Network Essay Series Teaching Excellence: Toward the Best in the Academy, vol. 9. Ames, IA: POD Network; 1997–1998.

Michaelsen LK, Black RH, Fink LD. What every faculty developer needs to know about learning groups. In: DeZure D, editor. To Improve the Academy: Resources for Faculty, Instructional, and Organizational Development. Stillwater, OK: New Forums Press; 1997.

Michaelsen LK, Black RH. Building learning teams: the key to harnessing the power of small groups in higher education. In: Kadel S, Keeher J, editors. Collaborative Learning: A Sourcebook for Higher Education, vol. 2. State College, PA: National Center for Teaching, Learning, and Assessment; 1994.

Michaelsen LK, Fink LD, Knight A. Designing effective group activities: lessons for classroom teaching and faculty development. In: DeZure D, editor. To Improve the Academy: Resources for Faculty, Instructional, and Organizational Development. Stillwater, OK: New Forums Press; 1997.

Michaelsen LK, Knight AB, Fink LD, editors. Team-Based Learning: A Transformative Use of Small Groups in College Teaching. Sterling, VA: Stylus; 2004.

Michaelsen LK, Parmelee DX, McMahon KK, Levine RE. Team-Based Learning for Health Professions Education: A Guide to Using Small Groups for Improving Learning. Stylus: Sterling, VA; 2008.

Michaelsen LK, Richards B. Drawing conclusions from the team learning literature in health-sciences education: a commentary. Teach Learn Med. 2005;17:85–8.

Michaelsen LK, Sweet M, Parmelee DX, editors. Team-based learning: small group learning's next big step. San Francisco, CA: Jossey-Bass; 2009.

Michaelsen LK, Schultheiss EE. Making feedback helpful. Organ Behav Teach Rev. 1988;13(1):109–13.

Miflin BM, Campbell CB, Price DA. A conceptual framework to guide the development of self-directed, lifelong learning in problem-based medical curricula. Med Educ. 2000;34:299–306.

Morrison G, Goldfarb S, Lanken PN. Team training of medical students in the 21st century: would Flexner approve? Acad Med. 2010;85(2):254–9.

Nieder GL, Parmelee DX, Stolfi AS, Hudes PD. Team-based learning in a medical gross anatomy and embryology course. Clin Anat. 2005;18:56–63.

Ortega RA, Stanley G, Snavely A. Using a media centre to facilitate team-based learning. J Vis Commun Med. 2006;29:61–5.

Parmelee D, Michaelsen L, Cook S, Hudes P. Team-Based Learning: a Practical Guide, AMEE Guide No. 65, 2012. Med Teach. 2012;34(5):e275–87. Epub 2012 Apr 4

Parmelee D. Team-based learning: moving forward in curriculum innovation. Med Teach. 2010;32:105–7.

Parmelee DX, DeStephen D, Borges NJ. Medical students' attitudes about team-based learning in a pre-clinical curriculum. Med Educ Online. 2009;14(1)

Parmelee DX, Hudes P. Team-based learning: a relevant strategy in health professionals' education. Med Teach. 2012;34:411–3.

Parmelee DX, Michaelsen LK. Twelve tips for doing effective team-based learning (TBL). Med Teach. 2010;32:118–22.

Pileggi R, O'Neill PN. Team-based learning using an audience response system: an innovative method of teaching diagnosis to undergraduate dental students. J Dent Educ. 2008;72:1182–8.

Poirer TI, Butler LM, Devraj R, Gupchup GV, Santanello C, Lynch JC. A cultural competency course for pharmacy students. Am J Pharm Educ. 2009;73:81.

Regehr G. Trends in medical education research. Acad Med. 2004;79:939–47.

Reznich CB, Anderson WA. A suggested outline for writing curriculum development journal articles: the IDCRD format. Teach Learn Med. 2001;13:4–8.

Searle NS, Haidet P, Kelly PA, Schneider VF, Seidel CL, Richards BF. Team learning in medical education: experiences at ten institutions. Acad Med. 2003;78(10 suppl):S55–8.

Seidel CL, Richards BF. A comparison of in-class learner engagement across lecture, problem-based learning, and team learning using the STROBE classroom observation tool. Teach Learn Med. 2005;17:112–8.

Seidel CL, Richards BF. Application of team learning in a medical physiology course. Acad Med. 2001;76:533–4.

Shankar N, Roopa R. Evaluation of a modified team based learning method for teaching general embryology to 1st year medical graduate students. Indian J Med Sci. 2009;63:4–12.

Shellenberger S, Seale JP, Harris DL, Johnson JA, Dodrill CL, Velasquez MM. Applying team-based learning in primary care residency programs to increase patient alcohol screenings and brief interventions. Acad Med. 2009;84:340–6.

Sweet M, Michaelsen L, eds. Team-based learning in the social sciences and humanities group work that works to generate critical thinking and engagement. Stylus; 2012.

Team-Based Learning Collaborative. www.tblcollaborative.org. Accessed November 17, 2011.

Thomas PA, Bowen CW. A controlled trial of team-based learning in an ambulatory medicine clerkship for medical students. Teach Learn Med. 2011;23:31–6.

Thomas PA, Bowen CW. A controlled trial of team-based learning in an ambulatory medicine clerkship for medical students. Teach Learn Med. 2011;23:31–6.

Thompson BM, Schneider VF, Haidet P, Levine RE, McMahon KK, Perkowski LC, Richards BF. Team-based learning at ten medical schools: two years later. Med Educ. 2007b;41(3):250–7.

Thompson BM, Schneider VF, Haidet P, Perkowski LC, Richards BF. Factors influencing implementation of team-based learning in health sciences education. Acad Med. 2007a;82(10 Suppl):S53–6.

Thompson B, Levine RE, Kennedy F, et al. Evaluating the quality of learning team processes in medical education: development and validation of a new measure. Academic Medicine. 2009;84(10):124–7.

Touchet BK, Coon KA. A pilot use of team-based learning in psychiatry resident psychodynamic psychotherapy sessions. Acad Psychiatry. 2005;29:293–6.

Varpio L, Bell R, Hollingworth G, Jalali A, Haidet P, Levine R, Regehr G. Is transferring an educational innovation actually a process of transformation? Adv Health Sci Educ Theory Pract. 2012;17(3):357–67.

Vasan NS, DeFouw DO, Compton S. A survey of student perceptions of team-based learning in anatomy curriculum: favorable views unrelated to grades. Anat Sci Educ. 2009;2:150–5.

Vasan NS, DeFouw DO, Holland BK. Modified use of team-based learning for effective delivery of medical gross anatomy and embryology. Anat Sci Educ. 2008;1:3–9.

Weiner H, Plass H, Marz R. Team-based learning in intensive course format for first-year medical students. J Educ Eval Health Prof. 2008;5:3.

Wiggins G, McTighe J. Understanding by design (Merrill Education/ASCD College Textbook Series); 1998.

Woolley AW, Chabris CF, Pentland A, Hashmi N, Malone TW. Evidence for a collective intelligence factor in the performance of human groups. Science. 2010;330(6004):686–8.

Zgheib NK, Simaan JA, Sabra R. Using team-based learning to teach pharmacology to second year medical students improves student performance. Med Teach. 2010;32:130–5.

Index